The Advantages of Nearly Dying

The Advantages
of Nearly Dying
Michael Rosen

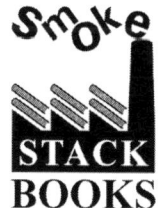

Smokestack Books
1 Lake Terrace,
Grewelthorpe,
Ripon HG4 3BU

e-mail: info@smokestack-books.co.uk

www.smokestack-books.co.uk

Copyright 2023,
Michael Rosen

ISBN 978-1-7397722-9-1

Cover image:
David Levene/
Guardian/eyevine

Smokestack Books
is represented
by Inpress Ltd

For Emma

Preface

How the government ended up killing and maiming us in February, March and April 2020.

On 3 February 2020, Boris Johnson made a speech in Greenwich:

'And in that context, we are starting to hear some bizarre autarkic rhetoric, when barriers are going up, and when there is a risk that new diseases such as coronavirus will trigger a panic and a desire for market segregation that go beyond what is medically rational to the point of doing real and unnecessary economic damage, then at that moment humanity needs some government somewhere that is willing at least to make the case powerfully for freedom of exchange, some country ready to take off its Clark Kent spectacles and leap into the phone booth and emerge with its cloak flowing as the supercharged champion, of the right of the populations of the earth to buy and sell freely among each other.'

(Translation: we governments shouldn't use the powers of the state to intervene against this virus because they will prevent the market from operating freely. So the virus should be allowed to fly free round the population, so that the market can be free. Mass death would be a necessary price to pay for the market to go on doing what it does – part of which is to produce the great inequalities we know of so well. And, irony, guess who would be high risk in the face of the virus? Those who experience the rough end of inequality, the poor. Could things have been stated more clearly and more horrifically than this?)

A further angle to take on this is that what Johnson is signalling here is along these lines: other countries will intervene to try to stop the virus but we won't; this means that we will have a competitive advantage over them.

This is a possible interpretation too.

On 3 March 2020 Boris Johnson said at a press conference:

'I was at a hospital the other night where I think a few there were actually coronavirus patients and I shook hands with everybody, you'll be pleased to know, and I continue to shake hands.'

Two days later he was interviewed on TV, where Philip Scofield asked:

'Is the delay [ie the attempt to delay the spread of the virus] essentially trying to spread this out so it doesn't all happen at once and overwhelm the NHS, and that you can actually delay it into perhaps the summer when it's a little bit quieter and the ordinary flu might have died down a wee bit, is that what you're doing?'

Johnson replied:

'Well it's a very, very important question, and that's where a lot of the debate has been and one of the theories is, that perhaps you could take it on the chin, take it all in one go and allow the disease, as it were, to move through the population, without taking as many draconian measures. I think we need to strike a balance, I think it is very important, we've got a fantastic NHS, we will give them all the support that they need, we will make sure that they have all preparations, all the kit that they need for us to get through it. But I think it would be better if we take all the measures that we can now to stop the peak of the disease being as difficult for the NHS as it might be, I think there are things that we may be able to do.'

(Note what Johnson is doing here is first stating the idea of Herd Immunity without vaccinations that scientists and others have told him. He does not, as has been stated, dismiss this totally. He modifies it in his terms: 'I think we need to strike a balance'. He is saying that trying to engineer some Herd Immunity without vaccination is OK but the government will also take 'measures' too. It's clearly a mixed message.)

On 12 March Robert Peston had his usual inside story in *The Spectator* with a headline 'Herd immunity' will be vital to stopping Coronavirus' and wrote of this desirable outcome without mentioning the inevitable huge loss of life involved nor the high chance of it being unachievable.

On 13 March, three government scientists sang the same tune. Graham Medley told BBC *Newsnight*, 'We're going to have to generate herd immunity... the only way of developing that in the absence of a vaccine is for the majority of the population to become infected...' Sir Patrick Vallance said on the *Today* programme, 'Our aim is to try and reduce the peak, broaden the peak, not suppress it completely; also because the vast majority of people get a mild illness, to build up some kind of herd immunity.' John Edmunds said, 'The only way to stop this epidemic is indeed to achieve herd immunity'.

These people were talking of engineering a situation in which mass death would take place. It's not as if science is unaware of the Black Death, Myxomatosis, Polio or Dutch Elm Disease – all with mass fatalities and maiming.

The extraordinary fact is that this idea of 'herd immunity' without vaccination is lousy biology. No one knew then how long or short nor how strong or weak the body's immune response would be to this virus. No one knew how often it would mutate nor how different the mutations would be from the original virus. These scientists were gambling with 'known unknowns' some of which would result in no 'herd immunity'.

What's more, the limited 'herd immunity' without vaccination that occurs naturally usually involves the evolutionary process of 'breeding out' (through death, before they reproduce) of those individuals who are susceptible to the virus and the 'breeding in' of those who are resistant, assuming the resistance is inheritable. This takes generations to effect – if ever. The problem for this scenario is that the section of the population most affected by the virus is above 'breeding' age! This negates the process by which evolution favours resistant individuals.

It seems to me horrific that top scientists were able to put forward their proposals to enact mass killing without being challenged, either on ethical or biological grounds. If you want to find out why or how this government has been lax, chaotic, incompetent and cruel in its approach to Covid-19, it starts here.

The consequence is that there have been tens of thousands of deaths, and there are tens of thousands of us with long term or lifetime debilitating consequences.

They must never be let off the hook.

Michael Rosen
2022

Contents

Ghost	17
Biblical	18
I Am Not Getting Better	19
I Forgot	20
Hospital	21
Cold	22
The Moment I Think I'm Gonna Get Busy	23
I Know I'm An Oldie	24
I Lost Seven Weeks This Year	25
I Am Not Who I Was	26
Alarms	27
Pain and Risk	28
The Good News	29
On TV	30
Dream	31
Ground Glass	32
Instead	33
More Alarms	34
Covid Took My Toenails	35
At the Chiropodist	36
I Woke Up	37
I Got Six Numb Toes	38
Talking to My Toe	39
Socks	40
I Squeezed My Toe	42
How is My Toe Doing?	43
Lucky	44
Update on the Toe	45
Renewal – a Soliloquy	46
My Days Are Measured Out in Eyedrops	48
I Did an Eye Test Today	49
Clint Eastwood	50
The Eye Clinic	52
More Good News	53
At the Eye Clinic	54
Waiting to Be Seen	55

Well Done	56
Forgotten	58
In the Vaccination Observation Room	59
In the Hospital	60
Holes	61
Good Result	62
Every Day	63
Actually	64
Dream	65
Whether	66
Hearing Myself Think	67
Switched On	68
Ain't Life Sweet?	69
Forgetting	70
Alcove	71
Hot	72
Mud	73
Voice Therapy	74
Spoon	75
My Hearing Aid	76
Tracheostomy	77
Ancestry	80
Balloon	81
Gesundheit	82
Actually	84
Klutz	85
As I Go to Sleep	86
Problems	87
Nureyev	88
Cold Hands	89
In the Morning	90
The Consultant	91
Mr Jacobs	93
Hospital	94
Heel	95
Microbleeds	96
The Brain Hospital	97
You Get Used to The Body You've Got	98

The NHS and the People	99
Scaly Monsters Emerge	100
It Was an Intimate Time	101
O Let's Do Away with the Oldies	103
Dick Whittington's Cat	104
Every Day	106
Very Moral	107
It Seems	108
Underlying	109
People	111
Mass Murder	112
The Dead Can't Speak	113
Foreigners	114
Herd Immunity	115
Anger	116
Choice	117
Where	118
Quote of the Year	119
The Curve	120
I Must Try Harder	121
Apparently	122
This Christmas	123
I Didn't Have Covid	124
They Say	125
Tough Call	126
Ceiling	127
The Vicious Narrative	128
The Peter Principle	129
I've Seen People Prepare for Funerals	130
J'accuse	131
The Past	133
Eddie: The Silence	135
Eddie: The Hardest Bit	136
Every So Often	137
If I Let Myself Think of Meeting Him	138
Two Days After He Was Born	139
Some Days	140
I Studied Meningitis	141

Every Year	142
There Are People in Their Forties	143
Death's Door	144
Eighteen Months After I Woke Up	146
Every Now and Then	148
While I Was Waiting for My Shingles Jab	149
Asides	150
Broadcasting	152
The Advantage of Having a Body	153
The Advantage of Nearly Dying	154
My Brain	155
At the Bank	156
Straight Lines	157
Worrying Moment	158
Weekends	159
Ghost	160
Directionality	161
The Great Thing	162
Article	163
Lonely Places	164
What's the Difference?	165
The House is Silent	166
Last Night	167
Doze	168
Prompt	169
No Words	170
Rehab	171
I Don't Understand	173
The Physio	174
While There's Time	175
Dissolution Street	176
One Great Reason for Cutting Overseas Aid	178
Contagious	179
To Save People the Bother	180
Over in the Right-wing Mags	181
Being Jewish	182
Sonnet for Anne Frank	184
Learning	185

As If in a Dream	186
If They Want To	189

Ghost

I wander about the streets of Muswell Hill.
People see me.
They say
'You're alive!'
I say,
'Am I?
How do you know?'
I think,
how DO I know?
How can I be sure?
Maybe I'm a ghost.
A Jewish ghost.
A Jewish ghost is called a 'dybbuk'.
They wander about haunting people.
I'm The Dybbuk of Muswell Hill.

The thing is
I tried to die
and they wouldn't let me.
So I'm probably alive.

Biblical

I was in a coma for forty days and nights.
It was a bit biblical of me.
I am Noah in the rain,
40 days and 40 nights
then sending out the dove
who came back with the olive branch
telling Noah the storm was over,
Miss Stafford telling us the story in assembly.
And then Jesus
Miss Mount,
telling us of Jesus in the desert
fasting for forty days
being tempted by the devil
but not giving in, living through it.
And Miss Mount again,
telling us of the 40 days
between the resurrection and the ascension.
(I was never sure what Jesus was doing for so long.)
Did my doctors use these biblical moments
as a guide?
Did they see me on an Ark
sailing through the rains?
Or was in the wilderness trying to resist and survive?
Or was I in some space between life and death
that they measured out for me biblically?

I Am Not Getting Better

at dropping eye drops
into my eye.
I miss my eye
as often as ever,
the drops hit my nose, my forehead, my temple...
This tells me
that learning is
not easy
and that 'practice makes perfect'
is a saying that is
not perfect.

I Forgot

I forgot Sean Connery's name earlier.
I've remembered it now.
It's Sean Connery.

Hospital

A nurse says to me,
'You must on no account get out of bed.'
I say, 'I won't. I can't. I can't even stand up.'
She says, 'but you tried to get out of bed last night.'
I say, 'I didn't try to get out of bed last night. I fell out of bed.'

Cold

Cold hands creep up on me.
Not yours. Mine.
As the day slows down,
the hands chill.
With hands like these
I could be trusted to cool drinks.
It's as if I had put them in the fridge
to set. Like jelly. Or a chocolate brownie.

I put them in my armpits
but this limits what else I can do.
It's difficult to type with my hands
in my armpits.
If I'm in an armchair
I put them under my bum
but there's not much point
being in a soft armchair
if you're sitting on bony lumps.

Running round the kitchen
can warm them a bit.
Why are you running round the kitchen?
To warm my hands up.

My mother's hands were cold.
Perhaps they're hers.

The Moment I Think I'm Gonna Get Busy

my body decides it wants to be dizzy
I stagger about, walk into chairs
grab the table, trip on the stairs
I'm dying for a pee, I really gotta go
Hold it. I daren't. I got vertigo.

I Know I'm An Oldie

but I didn't expect to go mouldy.
I got Covid last year
I thought it would clear
but they say my skin's in a state
where it will granulate.
It's something you see rather than feel
Look! I've started to peel...

I Lost Seven Weeks This Year

I lost seven weeks this year.
I'm looking for somewhere
where I can get
some replacement ones.

I Am Not Who I Was

I am not who I was.
Every day is a struggle
to not be sad about that.

Grief is being sorry
that things aren't the way they were.

Things not being the way they were
is grief.

Yet nothing is the way it was.

Even in grief
we see
that we are part of all things
becoming different.

Alarms

Alarms are great for
short term memory loss.
The alarm goes off –
it's a reminder –
then I say to myself,
'What did I set the alarm for?'

Pain and Risk

I read a lot about artists' pain.
For a while I was envious
because there didn't seem to be
much pain in Pinner.

Then I read a lot about artists' risks.
They came and told us about
what they saw when they risked
everything.
I decided that risk mattered
more than pain.
But I didn't risk anything.

Then I got ill
I got pain.
and it seems like I risked
everything I've got.
So now I don't envy anyone.

The Good News

Respiratory report:
my left ventricular ejection fraction
is normal.

Now I'm proud of my left ventricle.

On TV

On TV people are saying
there could be a gene that says to you:
if you get Covid, you'll get bloody ill.

I feel they're looking out of the TV
into my chromosomes.

Dream

There's a lonely corridor.
I'm lonely in the corridor.
The lonely corridor
connects with other corridors.
These are corridors
that I once walked down.
I have to go on down the lonely corridor
towards the other lonely corridors.
The lonely corridors up ahead
are corridors I've been down before.
They should be behind me.

Because they're up ahead,
it means
I can go along them.

I can't stop myself going along them.

I go along them.

Ground Glass

I've been looking at
my hospital discharge notes.
It's a post mortem.
Especially the bit about ground glass
in my lungs.
When did I put ground glass into my lungs?

Instead

Instead of Christmas decs this year,
I've bought a set of
rubber exercise bands.
Each of them comes
in a different (and lurid) colour.
Whenever I feel like I need a bit of yuletide joy,
all I have to do is get out a band,
give it a stretch and
(grunt)
I feel seasonal.

More Alarms

Each day
I set the alarms on my phone
to remind me when to take the eyedrops.
Today it's on the half hour every two hours.
For 15.30, I set it at 15.29 by mistake.
But I've left it as that
for the sake of variety.

I'm living wild.

Covid Took My Toenails

Covid took my toenails.
In their place were scabs.
The nails are growing
but one of them is growing into my toe.
I went to the chiropodist.
It's granulating, she said.
She put silver nitrate on it.

I read that in 1881
Carl Siegmund Franz Credé
introduced the use of silver nitrate
in newborn babies' eyes at birth
to prevent
contraction of gonorrhoea
from the mother,
which could cause blindness.

Fused silver nitrate, shaped into sticks,
was called 'lunar caustic'.

General Sir James Abbott
noted in his journals
that in India in 1827
it was infused by a British surgeon
into wounds in his arm
(resulting from the bite of a mad dog)
to cauterize the wounds
and prevent the onset of rabies.

Now my toe has history.

At the Chiropodist

I've been at the chiropodist.
Apparently one side of the nail
had grown in so far,
I had to have an anaesthetic
so that she could get the monkey wrench
and chain saw
down there to deal with it.

The bad news is
that it may not work,
so next time
she'll have to hack away
the two sides
with an axe and pour rat poison on it.

At one point she said,
'Got it. Look at this!'
and she showed me something like
a red carrot.
Apparently she had found it
in my toe somewhere.

I Woke Up

My big toes were numb.
Then the next toe on each foot
went numb.
Then the next.
Then the next.
I was worried that
my legs or arms
would go numb too.

Then everything.

I would have a numb head.

I Got Six Numb Toes

I got six numb toes
I got a peeling nose
that's how it goes

hey my skin grows
nodules in rows
that's how it goes

my fingers feel frozen
I feel I was chosen
that's Michael Rosen.

Talking to My Toe

I talk to my toe
I wish it well
I see its scabs
I look for its ooze
I poke it for pain
The new nail is in-growing

It's Covid calling
It nabbed the nail

And now the new one
echoes and calls me
back to the ICU bay
where I was
dead to the world.

Socks

One instrument of torture
that helped me to recover
was something called Ted socks.
One morning
they came to my bedside
and said that I had to wear Ted socks.
They said that when they had tried
to get me to stand up
all my blood
poured down into my feet
(I think that's what they said)
and it wasn't good.
It was stopping me being able
to stand up,
and if I wanted to walk
I had to start
by learning how to stand up.
Ted socks, they said,
would stop my feet
filling up with blood,
stop them stealing all the blood
meant for the rest of my body.
So they got me to lie down
and they levered my feet
and lower legs into Ted socks.
I remembered the video
of a crocodile snapping its jaws
round the leg of a buffalo
and hauling it into the river.
Three physios
cranked me up to a standing position
and propped me up
while the crocodile got to work
on my feet
and all the way up

to the bit just under my knees.
After I had been standing up
for about a year
(they said it was four seconds
and that I had done very well)
they let me lie down
but they said that I had to keep
the Ted socks on.
I lay in bed while the crocodile
carried on.
I was sweating
and the bite into my knees
was so bad I couldn't eat.
I pulled my legs up to my chest
dug my fingers into the top
of the Ted socks
and slowly peeled them off.
When they came back
the next day
to teach me how to stand up again
they saw that I had taken the Ted socks off.
They weren't pleased.
But they were kind
and didn't say that I had to.
They didn't refuse to teach me how to
stand up
just because I wouldn't wear the Ted socks.

I didn't ever ask them what Ted stood for.
I woke up this morning
and thought, what does Ted stand for?
Who is Ted?
Why did he invent those things?
Ted stands for:
Thrombo-Embolus Deterrent.
No wonder they hurt.

I Squeezed My Toe

and a blob of pus oozed out
from under the flange of skin
next to the nail.
Custard.
Beneath the skin
I could feel a hardness:
the nail growing sideways and downwards
out of sight
a tiny submarine
moving in the dark
against the innards of my toe.

I gave it intent:
'it' was doing this to 'me',
as if the 'it' wasn't 'me',
I disowned it,
so that I could feel it had picked on me
and attacked me.
I refused to think that it was my submarine
guided by me
into my toe-flesh.

How is My Toe Doing?

I haven't asked it,
because it's been dozing quietly
wrapped in a fur-lined condom.

Lucky

Lucky I cut the fronts off my crocs.
It means I don't exert any pressure
on my ingrowing toenails –
which hurt.

It also means that
when I do that crossing the leg thing
without looking,
I kick my toes against something,
there's nothing to protect me –
which hurts.

Update on the Toe

It got through the night
with no dressing on it.
Undressed, as it were.
This morning it had a shower
from my spray-on antiseptic.
'Freshened up'
as my mother used to say of the lettuce
as she dunked it in water.

Renewal – a Soliloquy

I took my two old feet to be checked out.
I was told my feet are as old as me
although it's fair to say the nails are new.

And there's the snag: last year I got Covid toes:
the big toe nails (the both), fell off in bed
I didn't see them fall, I was comatose
It's one way to spend six weeks I suppose.
I woke to see in place of nails, two scabs.

Alarmed, I showed my toes to those who came
to check, observe, and test my every move.
'They'll grow,' they said, and grow they did, o boy.
My toes, they chose, to grow both long and IN.
For fun, they dived in deep into the flesh.

I took my feet to those who deal with toes
out came the knives to probe, to trim, to cut.

But!

'Beware the skin,' they said, 'it's old, it's dry,
it thickens, cracks, reacts to nails in-grown.'
Disturbed by this, I asked: 'What shall I do?
D'you have meds, ointments, unguents or creams?'
'We have just that,' she said, 'a wonder cure.'

Aha, I thought, this must be something new
a great breakthrough in medical science.
'And what medication do you prescribe?'
I wondered, thinking of my future feet.
'Olive oil,' she said, 'Morning, noon and night.'

Olive oil? That's for salad dressing, no?
Frying herbs for spaghetti bolognese.
Artichoke hearts, dried tomatoes, hummus.
Really? On my toes? The soles of my feet?

Pro'bly best not to use the olive oil
that sits by the cooker in the kitchen.
So I bought a bottle just for my feet
not that I told them that in the shop
I didn't sidle up to the assistant,
and say 'Do you sell olive oil for feet?'

And so it is, each day, I wipe and bathe
my toes with golden green olive oil
my mind mulling on memories from school
the bible-stories, scripture, parables
the feet of people being anointed
and here's me: wiping, oiling my feet too!

I've been at it, some four or five weeks now
and what was old and dry and thick and cracked
where skin hardened under the ingrown nail
is now new and soft to touch or to stroke.

I could almost say that those toes are now –
thanks to olive oil – like a baby's cheek.
My toes may be old but I'm a new man.

My Days Are Measured Out in Eyedrops

One kind four times a day
Another every two hours.
Sometimes they coincide.
Sometimes they don't.
There's a pattern to this.
I can't do the maths.
Life is interesting now.

I Did an Eye Test Today

The operation on my right eye has enabled me
to see so well,
I can see through the hospital wall
into the car park outside.
The op on my left eye has stopped it bursting (glaucoma)
but it's still misty –
but not entirely so.
There's an inner circle
which is not-so-misty.
The vision in that eye
is as if I'm looking through a translucent bagel,
a bagel made of net curtains,
jelly-fish bagel.
Bagel-vision.

Clint Eastwood

Now that they've replaced my own lens
with a plastic one,
every day the view through my eyes is
different:
a new blur to my right
a brightened slash in the corner
and two trees where there was one yesterday.

At first
as I walked out the hospital door
it was all seasons of mists
without much fruitfulness
but perhaps that was the sticking plaster
over the transparent eye patch
making it not transparent
and the other eye is always Clint Eastwood anyway
playing misty for me.

As Vik the surgeon
took out my own lens
he said, 'Fat.'
We had looked at it on the scan
and I imagined it between his fingers
like a button
(I once cut a sheep's lens in half
in Biology)
and then he threw that bit of me
in a bin.
Unwanted spare part.

I stared at the arc lights
He called for a lens
and counted
1, 2. 3
as if it was going to leap from Petrie-dish
into the gaping hole of my eye.
I guessed he squeezed it in somehow.
I remembered drawing tiny muscles
thinning and thickening a lens.
I lay still, not daring to move
in case something missed.

And I wondered how those tiny muscles
connected to my new lens
or will it be as I imagined it:
a button in my eye
as inert as a magnifying glass?

I was good at not moving
though I gulped twice.

I should have asked to keep my lens.
I could have kept it in a jar of salt water.

What with all that Shakespeare in me
since I was ever,
I think of that shout, 'pluck out his eyes!'
and then: 'out vile jelly!'
If I could see it on the mantlepiece
in its jar
I wouldn't think it vile.
I might think of it like
a stuffed favourite cat
in its glass case.

The Eye Clinic

The good thing about the eye clinic is
that once they've checked
that you haven't got a temperature,
they give you a sticker.

My sticker says 'Tuesday'.
I stuck it to my jumper.
It's been there for a few days.
When people see me,
they'll know it's Tuesday.

More Good News

My eyeball is not going to burst.
Good news.
The drainpipes in my left eye
seem to be working.

At the Eye Clinic

A young man
with the disaster of a broken bottle
on his face.
A track round his mouth,
with a palette of bruises.

Waiting to Be Seen

Back at my new home: the eye clinic.
There are 65 eyes waiting to be seen.

Well Done

I sit down at the machine
again.
I know how it goes now.
I've been here forever
this year.
Look up, Mr Sharma says
and puts a drop in my eye.
I put my chin in the plastic cradle
my forehead against the plastic crescent.
He winches the apparatus higher.
He aligns lenses and lights
between my eyes and his.
Look down, he says
He lifts my eyelid.
He sighs.
He clacks about
Fetching something
that he clips on to the machine.
I stare towards blue lights.
It's a blurred street scene
at night.
I like it.
OK, he says.
I lift back from the machine.
14 and 17, he says.
That's good, isn't it? I say.
Yes, he says.
Is it draining? I say.
Yes, he says,
come back in a month.
Well done, I say.
No, well done you, he says.
Really? I think,
he did a micro-operation

inserting a tiny tube into my eye
and it's working.
All I did was turn up.

Forgotten

I've got Hollywood Stars Forgetting Syndrome
I forgot the names of big Hollywood stars:
Meryl Streep – forgotten.
George Clooney – forgotten.
Tom Cruise – forgotten.

In the Vaccination Observation Room

They're discussing Benedict Cumberbatch.
We wait for our timers to bleep.
The supervisor is waiting to see if we die.
The box for the timers
is called 'Used Timers'.

I ask them if they have one for 'Old Timers'.

In the Hospital

The therapist came to my hospital
to talk to me about eating.
The tracheostomy into my throat
could cause problems.
Things could get stuck.
I must always have some water
by me when I eat.
She told me of foods to avoid:
One of the foods was raisins.
I wanted to say to her:
But I am raisins.
You can't stop me eating raisins.
I tell children my name is
Michael Raisin.
Would it help
if we called raisins 'Rosens'?

When she went
She left behind a leaflet.
The leaflet said, avoid raisins.

I have disobeyed the instruction.

Holes

It seems like my appointment
for a CT scan is still on.
They need to look in my head
to see if anything's there.
Pretty sure there's some brain
but a few months after I came out of hospital,
there were some big holes.
I wonder if they've filled up.

Good Result

Bought new reading glasses yesterday.
Stronger.
Good Result.
Though it seems to have amplified the shadow effect of my left eye.
Emma comes in.
'Why have you got a sticker on your glasses?'
'Mm?'
I take the sticker off.
The shadow has gone.

Every Day

Every day I get up,
I check my left eye –
the eye is at its foggiest in the morning –
I put in my hearing aid,
I wiggle my toes to free up
a bit of the numbness –
all in the full knowledge
that it was Johnson, Cummings
and his incompetent unprincipled government
that caused this.

Actually

She asked me
what I had been doing.
I said, 'Trying not to die.'
I thought later,
actually, I tried to die
but they wouldn't let me.

Dream

I dreamt I was at a hospital
for cars.
I was taken down into the basement
and it was full of dead cars.
Thousands of them.
Like in a multistorey car park
but the cars were closer together.
It was a car morgue.

Whether

I seem to be doing more things than I can remember.
Emma tells me about something she says I said or did
and I have to decide whether

a) I can't hear her
b) I can hear her but can't remember
c) I can't hear and can't remember.

Hearing Myself Think

I've just discovered
if I turn my hearing aid up to max
I can hear myself think.
It's a squelching sound.

Switched On

Every morning I slot my hearing aid over my ear
push the soft plastic plug into my ear-hole
lay its tail into the curve of my ear
and switch on by snapping its tiny hatch shut.
Everything to my left,
a bird on the gutter, the kettle boiling, a tap running,
sounds as bright and tinny as speakerphone
on my mobile.
As I do this
I have a moment
where I imagine it will switch on my left eye too.
The numb fog will lift
and everything on the left side
will look garish
as if I've racked up the brightness control
on the TV.

Ain't Life Sweet?

When I'm bored or slightly anxious
I hunt for the tiny skin nodules
that grow on my back
and forehead
as a result of Covid.
When I poke them they fall off.
Then they grow again.
Always a mystery where.
Always fun to find.
Always fun to flick off.

Forgetting

Today I forgot the word 'antithesis'.
I guess the antithesis of forgetting
is remembering.

Alcove

Since I had a tracheostomy
I seem to have acquired a corner
a nook, or alcove
in my throat.
Small bits of food –
half a raisin, a vitamin pill
a ryvita fragment –
will head down my gullet
and then turn right
down a branch line
and hit the buffers.
It doesn't make me choke.
It seems quite comfortable
in there.
It's not exactly a tickle either.
Just a presence.
I'm not allowed to do the cough
that clears the throat
the NHS voice therapist said
I mustn't,
so I do vigorous swallowing
as if I'm flushing the loo
for the eighth time.
I also try to sponge it out
with a bit of soft bread.
My mother taught me how to do that
if a fish bone got stuck.
A fish bone?
Hah!
When was the last time
I saw a fish bone?

Hot

The American for 'hot flush' is 'hot flash'.
I only know this
because I get them
and looked it up online.
I don't know whether this is Long Covid,
a side effect of medication
or the menopause.
The menopause seems unlikely
but I don't know which sounds better:
flush or flash.

Mud

I've been trying to get away from
feeling precarious.
I do exercises:
squats, weights;
walking firmly
heels down first and hard.

I think it's a hoax.
I'm just trying to trick myself.
I'm play-acting at being who I was.

Beneath the surface
is Wobbly Man
who bumps into doors
and forgets which club Arsenal beat
last time Arsenal won the FA Cup.
It's not just that I look like
I'm walking on mud.
I'm thinking on mud.

Voice Therapy

Fiona the Voice Therapist
looks out of her zoom screen
and says that she can see
that I'm not using my diaphragm.
I say that it feels as if my voice is
reedy.
She is going to give me
semi-occluded vocal tract voice therapy.
She gets me to trill my lips
sing through my teeth
hum raspberries
and talk into my hand.
I offer *Frère Jacques,*
Twinkle Twinkle Little Star
and *Three Blind Mice*
as my exercise pieces.
I have to slur the notes.
'Glide up and down the scales.'
says Fiona.
She says that I should do
this before I go on the radio
or do a show for children.
There's good empirical evidence
she says
to show that semi-occluded vocal tract therapy
works.

Later
I sit in the loo
and hum raspberries
and sing *Three Blind Mice* into my hand.

Spoon

Bringing a spoon up from a bowl
to go into my mouth
is something I must have learned
when I was one.
For 74 years I've been good at it.
I can hardly think of a time
when I missed.
One-year-olds sometimes get distracted
as the spoon is half way between
the bowl and the mouth
and end up poking it into their cheek.
They often have a tray built into their high chair
so if the spoon offloads its cargo
they can pick it up later.
I do the same as the one-year-old missing
the mouth
but without the excuse of being distracted.
It's because my two eyes see different things.
I hadn't realised that
my eyes, though not looking directly at the spoon
as it approaches the mouth,
does in fact clock the spoon
and uses the information to make sure
that the spoon goes where it's supposed to go.
My problem is that one eye thinks
it's going in
and the other one thinks it's missing.
The result is that it does miss.
I'm not sure which eye is to blame.

My Hearing Aid

My hearing aid
amplifies sounds going on in my mouth.
'Don't gulp,' my 16 year old says.
'I'm not gulping,' I say,
'it's the hearing aid. It amplifies the sound
of me swallowing.'
He says, 'I don't care. Just stop gulping.'
'I could switch my hearing-aid off,' I say,
'but I might not hear what you're saying.'
'I don't care,' he says,
'don't gulp.'
I switch my hearing aid off.
'That's better,' he says.
'Mm?' I say.

Tracheostomy

I couldn't say the word
'tracheostomy'.
They told me that I had had a
tracheostomy.
When I lay in bed
I tried to remember the word.
I started with 'broncheo'
and 'bracheo'.
The hole in my neck
was covered in a plaster.
Every day, a nurse came
took the plaster off
and put on a new one.
I went home with it
and they told me a nurse
would come to the house
and change the dressing.
They did.
Every day
they changed the plaster.
I felt the cold of the antiseptic
on the hole.
I wondered if the hole
was big enough to look in.
Could they see my lungs in there?
Days went by.
Different nurses came.
It didn't close up.
They said it was 'granulating'.
I couldn't see it.
I didn't know what granulating was.
Whatever it was
it was stopping the hole closing.
One day at the eye clinic
I told the eye doctor.

He made a call.
A woman came from plastic surgery.
She was a very elegant Asian woman
who walked through the hospital corridors
as if they were in her house.
She walked ahead of me.
I said that I couldn't walk as fast as her
because I had been in intensive care
for 48 days.
She said, 'Really?'
I said, 'Yes'.
We got to her clinic.
It was a plastic surgery clinic.
I thought she was doing this
as a favour to the eye doctor.
There were no forms.
No one asked me for my date of birth.
When you're in hospital
people always ask for your date of birth.
She didn't.
Not once.
She said she would deal with the hole in my neck.
She got out some silver tools.
She told me that she was going
to put silver nitrate on it.
Then she stated cutting and snipping my neck.
She said, 'That would do it.'
I went home
wondering if the silver nitrate
would go down the hole
into my lungs.
It didn't.
The hole closed up.
I remember the word:
tracheostomy.
If I want to sound slick
I say, 'tracky'.
'A doctor put silver nitrate

on my tracky scar,' I say
'because it was granulating.'
I sound like I know
what I'm talking about.
I don't.
No idea at all.

Ancestry

I did a DNA test the other day.
The result came back
and it said
that I'm descended from a Jewish cobbler
living in Warsaw.
And a jelly fish.

Balloon

The occupational therapist
tells me to throw a balloon.
My mind tells me to throw the balloon,
but there's a gap between my head
and my feet.
There's nothing there.
I have lost everything from below my neck.
I am just a head.
I can feel that I had an abdomen.
My mind knows that I had an abdomen.
My mind can't make the abdomen work.
One part of my mind thinks
that I didn't have an abdomen.
That part of my mind thinks
if someone could come up to me
and put their hand on my abdomen
they would put their hand straight through me.

Gesundheit

Over fourteen years
I slowly puffed up.
My eyelids, fingers, lips puffed up.
I felt constantly cold.
My voice went gruff
My hair went wiry.
I slurred my speech.
My face was a white moon.
I slowed down.
I became a snail.

The doctor said it was my kidneys.
I went to the Renal Department
so that they could look at my kidneys.
The kidney doctor stared at me.
He said, 'I think that's a rubbish.
You're hypothyroid.'

I remembered 'hypothyroid'.
In the two years that I did medicine
about 16 years earlier.
There was a text book
and on the thyroid pages
there was a picture of a woman:
before and after.
Moon face, before.
Lean, bony face, after.
After treatment.
The kidney doctor got the students in,
'What's he got?' he said.
'Kidney trouble, sir.'
The kidney doctor blew up.
'Just because we're in the Renal Department
doesn't mean that his kidneys have failed.
Check his pulse, feel his skin, get him to talk!'

They did.
They didn't know.
'It's hypothyroidism!' he shouted.

He sent me to the Metabolic Unit.
They took some blood.
I came back a week later.
The Metabolic doctor was called
Dr Gesundheit.
(No one believes me when I say that
I had a doctor called Dr Gesundheit.)
I asked him how he got his name.
He said, 'Same as I got my genes.'
He opened my file.
'Technically, you're dead,' he said,
'your reading is so low, you should be in a torpor.'
He was American.
He said 'torpor' in a very American way.
He said, 'You have to come in now.
Really. It's urgent. You could pass out
at any moment.
You could be in a torpor.'
I was glad he said 'torpor' again.

I joined the Metabolic Unit.
I shared a ward with a boy who hadn't grown;
a man who found that some bits of him started growing
while the rest of him stayed the same;
a woman who had turned into a ball
well two balls, actually
her head and her body
and she had no neck.
They looked at me and said,
'You look bad.'

I thought
Technically, I'm dead.

Actually

I watched myself on a film about Intensive Care.
The consultant said
'We didn't know if Michael was brain dead.'
Didn't you? I thought,
well, I knew I wasn't brain dead.

Well no, actually I didn't know.

Well, actually actually
I don't know what I didn't know.

I don't even know what I did know.

And I don't know if I knew nothing.

Klutz

I was a *klutz*.
Not a big *klutz*
but something of a klutz.
Now
with my fogged eye
and fogged ear
I'm a big *klutz*.
When I put the plates in the cupboard
I miss.
I put the plate on a bowl.
When I type,
I press D instead of S
U instead of Y.
I put the paper over the back of the tray
of the printer
instead of in the tray.
Now I'm a big *klutz*.

As I Go to Sleep

I wonder if I will have to get up
in the night for a pee
and I think about the quiet dark
of the house
which will be there
if I do.

Problems

The problem with Long Covid
is that it's hard for people to call it 'being ill'.
Being ill was when we had 'the thing' –
whatever viral infection it was.
Then we 'got better'
or we 'recovered'.

If we have symptoms and conditions,
they're just 'problems' we are 'getting over'
or 'will get over'.

The words are a problem
because our family, friends
and some people in medicine
start to think we are just moaning
or exaggerating
or 'stuck'.

Nureyev

In order to remember
which pills I have or have not taken,
I play pill-box ballet,
dancing the boxes round the water glass,
their positions telling me the story
of what's done or not done.
In a way
I am Nureyev.
Though probably not.

Cold Hands

Always cold hands.
They said, That's low blood pressure, that is.
I thought of a lazy heart.
Not putting in the effort to pump blood
as far as my fingers.
The inner heat never gets out to the edges.
In hospital they said, Drink more water.
I drink more water.
I'm always drinking water.
Cold hands.
They said, walk about.
I walk about.
With cold hands.
I remember something:
my mother had cold hands.
She'd put them down my neck
to make me giggle.
I put my cold hands in my armpits.
I don't giggle.
In the history of the universe,
my cold hands don't have a big part to play.
They're not in the index of any major or minor works
on how society functions.
They don't matter.
They are cold though.

In the Morning

I wake up and wonder
if I got up in the night
or if that was the night before.
I re-run the legs swinging out of bed
the steps on the boards
the sit in the dark
the wait for the wee to stop
the up
the steps back
the sit on the bed
the leg-swing.

It happened.

But was it in this night
or the night before?

It doesn't matter.
I know it doesn't matter.
I don't want to be bothered
that I don't know
which night it was.

But to not know
is a sign of not lining things up;
of not having things in order.

I make it matter
though it doesn't.

The Consultant

The consultant says that I have scarring
on my lungs.
She tells me on the phone.
She has the scan in front of her.
I imagine a shadow
on a sheet of black and white plastic,
a dark crescent or an almost-black ink-blot.

She explains that it's a result of the blood clots
that once sat in the 'saddle' of my pulmonary artery.
They broke into bits which floated down
narrower and narrower pathways
into the smallest capillaries.
I'm guessing that if there are scars
there must have been a wound in there
and this scarring is how the body remembers.
I say 'the body' but it's 'my body'.
I should say 'it's how my body remembers'.
But then, my body is me.
Really, it's how 'I' remember –
except that I don't know it.
After all, my brain is not in my lungs.

I'd like to see the picture too
but it belongs to the consultant.
This whole thing has been about
people knowing more about me
than I do,
looking down my throat,
into my ear,
into my eye,
scanning my chest
making a map of my heart:
scopes, CTs, MRIs, echocardiograms.

What stories our insides tell them:
journeys down tunnels,
plumbing emergencies,
break-ins, attacks,
the slaughter of unwanted cells,
and their unnoticed deaths.
All I know are aches, sweats,
and swellings:
outside stuff.
These doctors
paint a painting that they can see
and I can't.
I just have words on the end of a phone:
clots, saddle, migrations, scars.

In bed, later,
I put my hand on my chest,
and close my eyes.

It's all in there.

It's the end of the story.

I remember her saying,
'I'm discharging you.'
And that's it.

Mr Jacobs

Nurse Joe kept a journal
of the time he was a nurse
 in the intensive care ward,
the ward where I was in a coma.

He sent it to me.
He changed our names.
I was Mr Jacobs.
He noted one day that even though
he knew Mr Jacobs was Jewish
he said a couple of Hail Marys for him.

Another day he wrote of himself
walking into the ward in the morning:
'Mr Jacobs is still alive.'

As I read this,
for a moment
I feel as glad as Joe that Mr Jacobs
was still alive.
Great - Mr Jacobs was still alive.
Then I remember – that was me.
I'm Mr Jacobs.
And I know I'm still alive because
I'm reading how Joe was glad
I was alive.

Then I realise
Joe cared that Mr Jacobs was alive.
And that's probably
part of why I am alive.

Hospital

I realise
I can't walk.

If I can't walk
I can't get upstairs.

If I'm in the kitchen
and I want a pee
I won't be able to get to the loo.

A month later
I come home.
We have a loo downstairs
next to the kitchen.
It was there all the time
hiding from my mind.

Later
I realise that it wasn't hiding.
It was stolen.
The coma stole the loo.

Heel

My mind talks to my body:
'Heel down first, heel down first.
Heel, heel, heel.
Don't do flat feet or your knees will hurt.'

The body doesn't talk back to the mind in words.
It talks with twinges, aches and pains
or with the comfort without them.

The mind feels the body.
The body doesn't hear the mind's words.
The body warns the mind.
The mind tells the body to do things.
The body keeps the mind informed
of whether it is doing the things
the mind tells it to do.

The mind is attached to the body.
The mind is in the head.
The head is part of the body.
The mind is part of the body.
Is the body in the mind?
I think so.

I walk across Ally Pally Park:
'Heel, heel, heel.'

Microbleeds

I had microbleeds in my brain.
So now I can't hear with my left eye
I can't see with my left ear
and I get muddled.

The Brain Hospital

At the Brain Hospital
they gave me a Cognitive Functioning Test.
The first question was:
'What is the name of the Prime Minister?'
I said, 'I know it, but do I have to say?'

You Get Used to The Body You've Got

You know it.
You may not have words for it
but you have pictures of bits of it
and how the bits move.
It says, 'Hi, I'm your back,
this is how I bend.
Hi, I'm your mouth
this is what your teeth feel like.
Hi, I'm your legs
this is how you walk.'
It's your body in your mind.
Then a big thing happens
and your body changes.
You've got a new body.
New body bits.
And your mind struggles to know it.
To start off with
it doesn't want to.
You don't want to know your new body.
You want your new body to go away.
Then,
slowly
you start to find out ways to
get to know it.
You can try not to though.
It won't make any difference:
it'll still be there, saying
'Hi, I'm your new body.'
It doesn't walk away.
It's always with you.
You have to get on together.

The NHS and the People

The NHS isn't an optional extra like a dry-cleaners.
The NHS is us.
From the cradle to the grave
it gives very nearly all of us the means to survive.
When people talk of 'the economy',
that's the people.
The people exist
because the NHS makes sure that we do.

Scaly Monsters Emerge

Scaly monsters emerge
from oceans and lagoons,
their shoulders sliming
across our cinema screens.

I emerged from a bed;
my bottom half as much use on land
as a mermaid's,
skin flaking into my vest
one eye on, one eye off
one ear on, one ear off,
brain spluttering like a clogged carburettor,
nodding wisely
to hide my miscues.

Can he live onshore? people asked.
I made an effort to adapt.
Learned the language.
Discovered there are others.
A number didn't live.
They are a number.

Most people are kind to the strangers.
Luckily, some say, luckily
the bed people were mostly old.

It Was an Intimate Time

It was an intimate time
but I don't know them.
Lying side by side
hardly wearing a thing
high on morphine,
tubes down our throats
drips in our arms
peeing down pipes
shitting on pads,
our bodies in the hands of others
We were waiting to survive
or die.
The space was arranged for 11,
one nurse for one bed
but there were 24 of us
so the one nurse ran between two beds,
sometimes more.
The PPE that turned up one day
was second hand,
the consultant said,
there was blood on it.
I got klebsiella
a bacterial pneumonia
that cavitates the lungs.
I think of it as scooping out the tiny caves
in there.
42% of us died,
the consultant said.
I make that as being about 10.
I don't know them.
I don't even know the survivors.
Once I was awake,
they took me somewhere else.
I didn't even know I had been in there.
If I was suspicious

I could think of it as
some kind of internment camp
that I wasn't awake to see
what they were doing to me.
I know now it's the only reason
I'm alive.
I've heard people say
that it's a scam.
Covid, that is.
Hashtag SCAMDEMIC.
Someone said on Twitter today
it's just a cough.
He said he doesn't know anyone who died.
I don't either
but I asked him if he had ever known someone
who's been murdered.
No, he said.
There you are, I said,
that proves that no one is murdered.

O Let's Do Away with the Oldies

O let's do away with the oldies
They take up too much space.
And who wants to be with an oldie
and look at their wrinkly face?

O let's do away with the oldies
O let's push them out of the door.
It's the rational thing to do
they're not productive any more.

Dick Whittington's Cat

Perhaps during Lockdown
some Number 10 partygoers
stumble out of the door
and throw drunken gags at each other
and one says,
'Hey, for a laugh, let's go find one of
these hospitals
where people are dying
and cheer'em up...'
and they stumble into cabs
and get to where Dick Whittington
heard the bells of London
where the Whittington Hospital looks out over London
and they manage to get the works lifts to work
they jam in
ride to the 5th floor
to the intensive care ward
where visitors are strictly forbidden
and they crash into the ward
cheering and laughing
'No need to bring your own booze
we've brought it.'
And they see us there
inert, plugged into tubes and lines
staring blindly
trying to live
and they say to us
'Hah! you think you're in a bad way?
What about us?
We're smashed.
It'll be hell in the morning
but what the fuck!
You're no bloody fun, are you?
Let's go, guys.'
And out they stream

out of the hospital
into the night street
and one of them finds
Dick Whittington's cat
in stone
a statue of a cat
on the pavement
and it becomes the funniest thing
that any of them have ever seen
It's a cat
it's a fucking cat
It's a statue of a fucking cat
and they have this great idea:
'Let's piss on it,' one of them says
And that's even funnier.

Every Day

Every day I get up,
I check my left eye –
the eye is at its foggiest in the morning –
I put in my hearing aid,
I wiggle my toes to free up
a bit of the numbness –
all in the full knowledge
that it was Johnson, Cummings
and his incompetent unprincipled government
that caused this.

Very Moral

If we live and then die
and that's the end
then there's no purpose
to life
other than life.
We're not saving things up.
There is just now.

That's why when governments wreck
the now
with wars and other calculated deaths
they destroy the only thing we have.
And there's no comeback for them.
They get away with it.
They're alive
and some of us are dead.

Some of them say sorry.
Mostly they don't.
Some are trained to say sorry
in a way that means
they weren't responsible.
The live on.
They are often in TV studios
talking about right and wrong.
They're always very moral.

It Seems

Viruses, like fish, have nationality.
The virus that's about to 'wash up on our shores'
(Johnson)
is presumably an illegal asylum seeker.
On the other hand,
the variant that first appeared in the UK
and has spread elsewhere,
Johnson calls just that:
a 'variant', just that,
so clearly, for him,
it's not acting illegally.
For him,
the UK variant doesn't 'wash up' anywhere.

This is 'science',
government style.

Underlying

They talked of 'underlying health problems':
Covid-19 was not really something
to be too bothered about
unless you had these underlying health problems.
As people with underlying health problems
were going to die soon
(they seemed to be saying)
then we really shouldn't get too bothered
about Covid.
We were given a picture
of perhaps just a few people
at death's door with terminal cancer
and the like.
And these people aren't your loved ones
and they aren't you
so relax.
Ignore them
and ignore Covid.

But the phrase didn't just refer
to people like this.
All sorts of people were
more likely to be affected by Covid:
a whole raft of possible susceptibilities.
And it's even affected some
who didn't seem to have any
underlying health problem.
Young women who run marathons
cropped up in the newspapers,
their lives massively altered by Covid,
struggling to climb stairs.

Talking of underlying health problems
was a way of dismissing Covid
as not really a problem for all of us.
Or more:
it was handy for
blaming people for getting Covid.
Covid was no longer a problem
for all of us.
It was just a problem
for near-dead people,
their lives thankfully shortened.

In fact
we all have underlying health problems
at some time or another.
Underlying health problems is us.
Life is an underlying health problem.

People

Johnson says that all schools must open,
but this will spread infection
so people have got to stay indoors.

He must think school students and teachers and school workers
aren't 'people'.

Mass Murder

Mass murder is mostly invisible
when governments do it.
They specialise in vanishing it:
indexing it under 'Operational difficulty'.
They can rely on news organisations
to look the other way,
make a fuss about a dead dog
or weep and forget.

The Dead Can't Speak

I can't speak for the Covid dead.
They can't speak.
When you ask me to come on the radio
or because you want to put me in your papers
I will say that I nearly died
because in February and March
the government failed to protect me
failed to protect all who've survived
and all those who have died.

Foreigners

There's a really dangerous virus coming from foreigners.
This from people who did nothing at all
in January, February and early March,
people governing a country
that's 'produced' millions of carriers
of the virus, some of whom
take it to other countries.

Herd Immunity

You aimed
but just missed
you with your bullets of
'herd immunity without vaccination'.
We were the necessary targets
the deaths without which herd immunity
you said
would not happen.
Many hit the target.
Dead.
You got me but not quite near enough
to heart or brain or lungs
to finish me off.
So now I'm here.
I see what you did.
I tell people what I saw
and heard.
You sat in your offices
and imagined that there were
acceptable levels of death.
You imagined that a virus
going through a population
would mean that everyone else
would be immune
without knowing for how long
or for how much of an immunity.
The whole thing was a gamble.
You gambled with our lives.
We lost.

Anger

The government diced with death.
Death won.

Choice

They gave us a choice:
people's freedom
to not mask, distance and wash,
versus our deaths and lifetime damage.
They went with 'freedom'.

Where

Where is the mentality produced
that sits in government committees,
tv studios and labs
juggling with hundreds of thousands of lives
in wars or pandemics?
What kind of training
makes them think of humanity in that way?

Quote of the Year

'Not to put too fine a point on it, from an entirely disinterested perspective, the Covid-19 might even prove mildly beneficial in the long term by disproportionately culling elderly dependents.'

Jeremy Warner
Daily Telegraph
3 March 2020

The Curve

For the last 24 hours,
scientists have been searching for
the 'curve' that Priti Patel says
that we are 'ahead of'.
If you are able to find it,
please ring our Helpline.

I Must Try Harder

I must try harder to understand
that I got ill
for the sake of the general good.

Apparently

If you have
'underlying health problems'
and you die
it doesn't matter as much
as people dying
who don't have underlying health problems.

This Christmas

'This Christmas,
we're going to suspend traffic laws.
It's up to the individual
as to whether you drive on the right or left
or whether you stop at traffic lights.
Happy Christmas.
Be sensible.'

I Didn't Have Covid

I didn't have Covid.
It's all a mistake.
I've been
in a second-hand bookshop
and said to someone,
'I've got Ovid'
and it all snowballed from there.
Sorry about the misunderstanding.
There are thousands like me.
All with copies of Ovid,
saying, 'I've got Ovid'.

They Say

They say:
If you collect together
in large gatherings
you'll get in trouble.

They say:
If you refuse to collect together
in large gatherings
(called 'schools')
you'll get in trouble.

Tough Call

Tough call:
do I believe a keyboard soldier
or people with years of study and practice
with viruses?

Keeps happening to me.
I ask the guy on Twitter
(who's been saying it's all a hoax),
whether he's a virologist,
and he says to me back, 'Are you?'

Ceiling

We had a teacher at school who said,
it's really scary
when you hit your intellectual ceiling.
I hit it tonight: trying to understand
what a politician was saying on *Newsnight*
Not a thing. Not a word.

I couldn't figure out
if he was in favour of what he got,
or of what he didn't get,
or of what he would like to get,
or of what he had no hope of getting
but still thought he would get
or even if he was in favour of
what he didn't want.

The Vicious Narrative

The vicious narrative is the one
that leaves us saying,
'What did I do wrong to have got Covid?'
rather than,
'what did the government not do that meant that I got Covid?'

The Peter Principle

The Peter Principle is
promoting people to their level of incompetence.
We need another 'principle'
to describe people being promoted to a level of amplification
of their irrelevance.

I've Seen People Prepare for Funerals

I've seen people prepare for funerals.
Sometimes they've asked me
if I had any thoughts on how to do them.
I say, 'Make sure, if you can,
that nothing will happen at the funeral
that will make you
sad or angry.
A funeral should be a good funeral.'
I thought there were things wrong
with my mother's funeral
and there were things that made me
sad and angry.
I thought that everything was right
for my son's funeral.
It was a good funeral.
People now are remembering
funerals at the time of
what look like governmental parties,
jollies in the garden.
They are remembering
mothers or fathers dying alone,
empty funerals
online funerals
lonely funerals.
They're not good funerals.
A funeral should be a good funeral.

J'accuse

thanks to Kevin Ovenden

a government of not protecting us

a government of experimenting with its population

a government of putting profit before people

a government of toying with the idea of 'herd immunity' without vaccination

a government of knowing that herd immunity without vaccination inevitably necessitates the deaths of hundreds of thousands of people

a government of knowing how little they knew about how Covid-19 works and that how it might spread, mutate, reinfect were unknowns and therefore any idea of 'letting it rip' was lethal and fatal to thousands of people

a government of refusing to listen to World Health Organisation guidelines issued from February 2020

a government of dishing out contracts to friends and supporters to provide services and equipment

a government that turned away from the local public health bodies that were best placed to run services

a government that has not provided and is still not able to provide a proper test-trace-isolate system which could and would protect more of its citizens

a government that decanted thousands of old people out of hospitals into care homes without them being tested, resulting in tens and thousands of deaths

a government of failing in early March to issue strict guidelines about social distancing, mask-wearing and hand-washing

a government of underfunding the NHS for ten years prior to the pandemic so that it was not sufficiently equipped to cope with the emergency

a small group of scientists of peddling the idea of 'herd immunity' without vaccination as a viable and ethical policy even though they knew that it necessitated the deaths of hundreds of thousands of people

journalists and commentators in major papers and news outlets peddling the idea that people over 70 were or are superfluous, unworthy of saving, who, if dead, would help the economy by not existing

journalists and commentators for helping to provide a seed-bed for what is in effect a form of creeping fascism, that a whole section of the population can be dispensed with for what is deemed to be a greater good.

The Past

I wonder how I manage to walk about
with Eddie dead inside me.
I've turned scenes into words
and put them on the page:
the morning bedroom
the arrival of men in uniform
the body bag sliding down the stairs.

There's a moment in the cemetery in Montparnasse
a woman sobbing by a grave,
I had thought that it must be recent
but she told her son had died years before
and she, poor woman, was adrift
drowning or drowned in her sorrow
and I hoped that wouldn't be me
in the years to come.

I worked long hours on finding out
about meningitis.
It was like fixing co-ordinates
on a point on a map:
its exact whereabouts in the landscape
of our biology.
I dwelled on how we live with bacteria,
how bacteria live with us,
how there are moments when organisms
cross frontiers
and find the beautiful, food-rich, warmth
of our blood.

I was never alone.
I've never been alone.
People tried hard
to stop me drowning.
And – look –
Emma and then two children.
Should I tell them that they saved me?
Now I have.
Does that sound as if that's what they're for?
To save me from falling into a pit
and not for what we made together?

Eddie: The Silence

The silence after lasts forever
Quieter than a painting.
There is nothing as quiet as this.
It is as quiet as nothing.

Eddie: The Hardest Bit

The hardest bit
is remembering him talking about
the things he wanted to do.
He was going to be a comedy chef, he said.
I see him in a TV kitchen
making his hot guacamole
and doing his matzo balls jokes.
He wrote a play
and asked me to help him put it on.
I did
but that was after he had died.

Every So Often

when he was growing up
I used to have a dream
where I'm in the water
with all the children
and we get into difficulty.
There's a raft,
I'm pushing them out of the water
on to the raft
but I can't get all of them on,
I turn round and I catch sight of a face
struggling,
and I realise it's Eddie.

If I Let Myself Think of Meeting Him

he never turns up.
We used to meet
at Ed's Diner
(it was named after him, we'd say),
or by the side of the theatre
where he was 'crewing'.
I go there in my head
but the road is empty.
The high windowless theatre walls
stretch upwards;
the stage door
where he would have bundled out
with his jacket not quite big enough
is quiet.
I wait.

Two Days After He Was Born

he slowed down,
became still.
The doctor said he had an infection
and the next 24 hours were critical.
I had to go home.
I lay there on my own
in misery,
sure that he would die.

Some Days

Some days I thought
it was my fault that Eddie died.
I didn't spot meningococcal septicaemia.
I didn't see it.
I thought
if it was my fault
i must have killed him.

I pore over stories of survivors of meningitis and meningococcal septicaemia.
Looking for something.

I Studied Meningitis

I started using the word 'bacterium'.
I read about meninges.
I got it that many of us walk about
with this bacterium
but we're not ill with it.
I got it that the problem is when
it crosses the membranes in our throat
and gets into the blood.
The bacterium multiplies in that environment,
breaks down membranes,
till our insides turn to 'mush'
the doctor told me.
'He wouldn't have known,' he said.

I think myself into his head
drifting off to sleep,
It's 2021 – 22 years later –
and I'm trying to capture his last thoughts
as if I'm pulling film out of an old camera.
I imagine flashes,
something dazzling
falling stars falling
night.

Every Year

the guys who he played hockey with
meet up.
They call him Big Eddie
and I hear stories
of how he kept the team bus amused
with jokes that even now,
over 20 years later
they'd rather not repeat.
There's talk of booze
and I twitch,
worried for a moment
that it was this that made him vulnerable?
Why did the bacterium 'decide'
that night to cross the membrane
in his throat and get into the blood?
What part of his make-up or life caused that?
I don't like it that there are no answers
for that, yet.
The guys play a game of hockey.
They beg me to get out there
and have a go.
My youngest does.
He zips about and the guys
men now of course
laugh and cheer him on
and I see them as they were
boys in that London Hockey final
they so nearly won
while Eddie, massive,
padded up in goal
did all he could to keep the ball out.

There Are People in Their Forties

who came as teenagers
and saw him
lying in a coffin
surrounded by flowers
in my front room.
I wonder if they've ever seen a dead body
since.

Death's Door

'You were at death's door.'
they say.
What is this door?
I know about the man
in the monk's outfit.
We can't see his face
and he carries a scythe
but he doesn't turn up with a door.
Where is death's door?
What does death's door look like?
I used to stare at the doors
of the suburban houses
where we lived.
I always thought
that when I walked past those houses
along the suburban streets
that the rooms were dark,
and the people inside
were sitting in the dark
or had died.
It was because no one was
allowed in the front rooms.
When I went over to see my friends
the mothers would say
don't go in the lounge.
And we didn't.
Though once my friend Harrybo
was allowed to take me in for a few minutes
to look at their new radiogram.
It was like a sideboard
but inside was a gramophone
and on the front was a radio
which lit up in an alluring way
and there were dials
which we twiddled

before our time in the lounge
came to an end.
Harrybo's house was called 'Merok'
and it was written up in the glass
over his door.
The door itself had a stained-glass panel in it
which cast an orange and blue light
into the front passage of their house.
We didn't have a front door
because we lived in a flat over a shop.
Our door was at the back of the building
next to the door to the shop.
It was dark green
with two frosted glass panels
which if you looked at from inside
when the co-op milkman called
for the bill
you could see a dark shape
behind the frosted glass.

Eighteen Months After I Woke Up

Eighteen months after I woke up,
I went to the Queens Square hospital
to have a brain scan.
After a day of tests
(bloods, blood pressure, echocardiogram,
cognitive functioning and a brain scan)
I was taken to a small room
to meet the consultant.
He said, 'Do you want to look at your brain?'

I thought about that.
Do I want to look at my brain?
I've been trying to look at my mind
for the last 50 years,
maybe I'll see something new.

I said yes
and he put up a slide on his screen.

It was a cross section of a cauliflower.
'It looks like someone who had altitude sickness,' he said.
I felt sorry for the cauliflower.
'You had micro haemorrhages,' he said.
I felt even more sorry for the cauliflower.
I wondered what my mind made of
being showered with tiny splashes of blood.
I studied the slide.
I couldn't see the micro haemorrhages.
'They're all cleared up now,' he said.

Now I thought of a brain mop,
going round cleaning up blood.

I had better not say any of this, I thought.
I stared at the screen.
I remembered what I was thinking about
when the machine was scanning my brain:
I was concentrating on a new way of breathing.

I'm looking at a brain
that is thinking about a new way of breathing,
I thought.
Shall I say that?
No.

Maybe one day
clever people like him
will look at the screen and be able to say,
'When we took this one,
you were thinking about a new way of breathing,
weren't you?'
In the meantime
I'll bear in mind
that he knows a lot about my brain getting showered
with blood.

Every Now and Then

Every now and then
I get the memory of the hospital smell again.
A déjà-whiff.

I'm beginning to think
I'm attached to hospital now.
My head lives there.

While I Was Waiting for My Shingles Jab

today at the docs,
I checked my blood pressures
and googled them on my phone.
First site that came up
bunged up an ad
before I could check them.
It was for insurance for funeral costs.

Asides

The physio is glad to see the back of me.

'Are you a haematologist?' I said.
'Bloody right I am!' she said.

The moment he looked me in the eyes
I knew he was an ophthalmologist.

My chiropodist footed the bill.

I exaggerated.
The radiographer saw through it immediately.

The surgeon who worked on my thorax
had a lot to say.
He needed to get it off my chest.

I was getting angry and my trichologist said,
'Keep your hair on, pal!'
And I said, 'No, you keep my hair on.'

I was late for my appointment
at the dentist.
I got there just in time
sat down in the chair
opened my mouth.
He looked in.
'You made it by the skin
of your teeth,' he said.

My pathologist is having problems.
He's on the slide.

My echocardiographer said he was in a hurry.
He could feel the pressure.

Had to go to Barnet Hospital.
Hair problems.

My dietician said
that I should try to look at the problem
organically.

My dermatologist asked me
why I was meddling in something
that was nothing to do with me.
He said, 'You've got no skin in it.'

She was from Critical Care
and said
she thought
that the recent production of *King Lear*
wasn't quite as good
as it should have been.

Have arrived early
at Ophthalmology department.
Can't see anyone.

There were a lot of visitors.
Matron was trying to ward them off.

Broadcasting

Back doing broadcasting.
Loving it.

It would have been hard to do
if I had died.

The Advantage of Having a Body

The advantage of having a body
working at about 50%
and a brain at about 90%
is that the brain makes up
for the body's incapabilities.

The Advantage of Nearly Dying

The advantage of nearly dying
is you get to see ahead of time
which people will think kindly of you.

My Brain

I don't think they're too worried about my brain.
My appointment for my scan
has been postponed from next Thursday to next year.

At the Bank

Someone can't be bothered
to stick to the lanes
laid out to keep us separate.
The NatWest doing its best
to make it less likely we'll breathe
on each other.
She walks into me as if I'm in her way.
I wait.
I glance down at the table to one side.
It's a picture of Vishaal.

They told me about Vishaal a few weeks ago:
Caught Covid same time as me
got over it.
got a stroke
and then died in June
months later than the 28-day limit.
He won't appear in the stats.
Here he is, smiling
In his NatWest uniform
Just like when he and I
traded gags about his Spurs
and my Arsenal.
He wasn't long married.
They had just bought a house.

Straight Lines

In my life there have been straight lines.
They seem to last about 5 to 10 years.
Then the straight line comes to an end
And there's big wiggle.
The line goes all over the place.
It's as if my pen hit something on the page
And goes off in several directions.
This lasts for 2–5 years and then it
Settles down again for another 5–10 year straight line.
So far, the wiggles have been moving school, deaths, diseases and divorces.
Moving school and divorces are just as they sound.
Nothing to add.
Deaths: my parents, my son.
Diseases: hypothyroidism, Covid-19.

Worrying Moment

Came back from the shops,
dug round in cupboard for my crocs,
put them on, walked round the kitchen.
I seemed to be more lopsided than usual.
What's happened?
Did stretches.
Still lopsided.
Sat down.
Glanced at crocs.
They weren't a pair.
Odd crocs.

Weekends

The weekend
doesn't end the week anymore.
It's either all week.
Or all end.

Ghost

People keep making the mistake
of thinking I'm alive.
They say things like,
'Nice to see you.'
Years of Hollywood movies
and they still don't believe in the paranormal.
I'm a ghost.
Get over it.

Directionality

I'm on my own downstairs.
Upstairs: a full house.
There's a noise.
I think it's away to my right,
possibly behind me.
It could be the pipes creaking.
Rain on the glass roof.
Magpies laughing.
Squirrels arguing.
I'm really not sure
if it's to my right or to my left.
I'm not really sure
if it's behind me or through the door.
I've lost something I'll call
'directionality'.
I don't think it matters
whether it's pipes, rain, magpies or squirrels.
My life doesn't rely on it.
I'm on my own downstairs.
Upstairs: a full house.
There's a noise.

The Great Thing

The great thing about
doing my exercise laps
round the block
is that I discover a new shop
each lap that I do.
Last time I think I saw
a charity shop in aid of people
with odd shoes,
a gift shop for men over the age of 109,
and a shop that sells keys that don't fit.

Article

There's an article about me
in the Waitrose *Weekend* newspaper.
I look like I'm nearing my sell-by-date.
I should have a yellow label stuck on me
with 'Reduced' written on it.

Lonely Places

When I came home
I pretended I was happier than I was.
I pretended that
I wasn't finding myself
back in the lonely places
of the hospital
again and again.
Sometimes the lonely places
join up,
lonely places in the hospital
lonely places before the hospital
lonely places since the hospital.
Every time this happens
I pause,
I look at it,
turn it over,
name it,
and try to drain it of its power to reach into me.

What's the Difference?

What's the difference
between what you were like
before you were ill
and since you were ill?

Before I was ill,
I thought I knew what I could do.
Since I've been ill,
I don't know what I can do.

The House is Silent

It's early.
I hear myself breathe.
The house is silent.
But something shifts.
A slight creak.
More silence.
Then another.
I remember yesterday.
We found two or three large spiders.
Someone explained
that September is the spider season.
How do they know? I wondered.
Do they talk about it?
'Here we go, September, again. In we go.'
Perhaps that shifting noise
is the spiders, I thought.
They're moving the furniture.
'Never did like that chair being so close to the window,
Dave, let's move it into the alcove.'
The house is silent.
It's early.
Something shifts.

Last Night

Last night
I died of a heart attack.

I knew it was a heart attack
because
1) it hurt,
2) because when I got Covid
   I got blood clots
   and blood clots cause heart attacks
3) because I had just had
   the booster jab
   which some people are saying
   can cause heart attacks
4) because when my father
   had a heart attack
   they told him at first
   it was indigestion
   but it wasn't indigestion
   which proved that this wasn't
   indigestion,
   it was a heart attack
   like my father's heart attack.

In the morning
the heart attack had gone.
I remembered that I did eat
an apple crumble with custard
with added giant sultanas
quite late
and it is possible that I ate it
quite quickly.

Last night
I died of a heart attack.

Doze

A doze crept up on me,
took me upstairs,
shoved me under the duvet
and shut my eyes.

Prompt

I was on a bus when two people sitting behind me started to talk to me. I said I lived nearby. They said they did too. I said that I had lived here when I was young. They said they hadn't lived here long. They had met while they were doing a play. I asked them if they were actors. Oh no, they weren't actors. They were just in a play. Well, said one to the other, you were in the play and I was the prompt.
'Really?' I said, 'did you do prompting every night when the play was on?'
'Oh yes,' she said.
Then the other one said, 'And then we were in another play and she had a part and it was me who did the prompting.'
'Did you ever have to actually prompt?' I said.
'Yes,' she said, 'she forgot a line to do with the radioactivity of a toaster.'
'And one night you forgot something too,' she replied.
'I don't think so,' she said back.
'Yes, the thing with the man next door who used to do weightlifting.'
'No, when you prompted, you dived in before I said it. I was trying to do a new pause.'
'I don't think you'd have got to the right words.'
'I would have. I know I would have. I know what I was thinking. You don't.'
'I think you think you know what you're thinking – which is a different matter.'
'There are times when I would like to have a prompt,' I said.
It was that moment in the day in winter when the lights of the shops start to be brighter than the light outside.

No Words

Today, they ask me what was it like
after I woke up
but I didn't have words then
to say what had happened to me
so I can't find words now.

There were words coming at me:
sedated, intensive care, ventilated,
intubated, tracheostomy.
Those words didn't say
why I was where I was.

I wanted
words for the muddle I was in
and the muddle was because
I didn't have the words.

They put me in a geriatric ward.
One nurse said to me,
'What are you in here for anyway?'
and I said,
'I don't know.'
And I thought
if I don't know
and you don't know
what am I going to do?

Rehab

In the Rehab Hospital
I tried very hard to be happy.
This Covid has hit me bad, I thought
but these people are trying to make me better.

One time
Emma and the kids
sat with me outside in the garden
and I told them I was doing OK.
We laughed in the sun.

She explained to me
that I had been in a coma.
You were in a coma for forty days,
she said,
they put you in a coma,
she said.
I said yes.

The next time they came,
a week later,
Emma told it to me again.
Was I? I said.
Yes, she said, I told you.
Yes, I said, as if I remembered.

I thought about Covid.
That was the bit I understood.
I knew I had had Covid.
That was why I couldn't walk
I thought,
but I was learning to walk
and I was doing OK
I thought.
Now, 18 months later

I see me back then
trying hard to be happy
but inside there were dark corners
where I was afraid that I had fallen apart:
the man who forgets yesterday.

I know now
that I couldn't walk
because I had been in the coma
for all that time.

If I want to confuse myself –
terrify myself even –
I try to remember
what it was like in that time
when I didn't know
that I had been in the coma.

I try to remember the next bit:
the feeling of not understanding
what Emma told me
and not remembering
what Emma told me.
And the next bit after that:
the long blank
where all I know is the word
'coma' but not the coma itself;
the long emptiness
the long muddle;
and it feels pathetic
that I tried so hard to be happy.

I Don't Understand

I talk to the self who was in the Rehab Hospital
18 months ago.
'Why do you think you can't walk, Michael?'
'I don't know. I think it must be Covid.'
'No, it was because you were in a coma for forty days.
You were in intensive care for 48 days.'
'Was I?'
'Yes. Emma told you.'
'Did she?'
'Yes, she told you that being in bed all that long
has 'deconditioned' you.'
'And that wasn't Covid?'
'No, listen: Covid's taken away your eye and your ear;
it's made you a bit breathless and a bit dizzy
but Covid isn't stopping you
from being able stand up or walk.'
'I don't understand.'
'You don't now but you'll get it after you leave here.'
'Is that where you're talking from?'
'I'm on the outside, at home, yes.'
'I will get home, will I?'
'Yes.'

The Physio

I said to one physio at the rehab
that I didn't think I would be able
to do a show
to 100s of children in a theatre again.
She said I would.
This year,
I did a show to 100s of children
at the Queen Elizabeth Hall.
A woman with her kids
asked me to sign a book.
It's me, she said.
It was the physio.

While There's Time

I take it that there is no purpose.
There's no design,
not one for all of us
not one for any single one of us
not one for me.
It is all pointless.
It's not even that this or that thing has more point
than anything else.
We are left with being here.
That's it.
That means being here
has to have purpose.
This year, this month
this week, this day
this minute.
It could be profoundly sad
that there is no overall purpose,
or design.
Lonely, purposeless creatures
floating through the universe.
Or it could profoundly encouraging
that what we have is being here
because we could make the best of it
while there's time.

Dissolution Street

after Bob Dylan's Desolation Row

The King is in the counting house, eating bread and money,
He thinks if he talks like Julius Caesar, we'll think that he is funny.
Plato has found a way to play chess, using tanks and guns
'Who cares?' says Henry Ford, 'we'll make ten thousand suns.'
John and Yoko close the curtains and get beneath the sheets
They can hear the bombs outside, falling on Dissolution Street.

The banker says to the poor man, 'You're helping keep things great.'
An unborn baby arrives in hell and says 'Sorry I am late.'
Louis Braille's lost his sight and says people keep giving him bad looks.
They say they know how to handle him, they take away his books.
King Midas tells the multitude there's always plenty to eat
The queue at the food bank stretches down Dissolution Street

They found that the judge was lying, so the judge changed all the rules
They found gold beneath the playgrounds, so they sold off all the
                                                                                      schools
Doctor Death went to hospital, where he met up with Dr Who
Doctor Death said he was out of cash, so he sold the hospital too.
The Sheriff of Nottingham was saying that it was honest to cheat
As he strung up Robin Hood on the gibbet on Dissolution Street.

The doctor's telling me the good news, my foot won't be falling off
The nurse is telling me I've got no lungs so I don't need to to cough.
Another nurse is telling me, 'Move!', cos I often fall out of bed.
The doctor's telling me more good news, he says I'm not brain dead.
The diary's open on yesterday but I don't know who I'll meet
They say I'm deconditioned, now I'm on Dissolution Street.

The Queen says that it's awful how people resent her fur coats.
The real problem she says is people arriving in small boats
They will eat every one of you, she says to you and me
The safest thing for all of us, is if we push'em into the sea
One or two can come ashore and as some kind of treat
They can be nurses or clean the floors in Dissolution Street

From the other end of the corridor, I hear a woman scream
I lean out of bed and ask the nurse, 'Can I stay in my dream?'
He says, 'You're dead anyway, so you're missing the bad weather.
This is the last place on earth where we're all working together.'
They bring in the last machine they have, I could see my heart beat
I might be dead now, I think, but we can leave Dissolution Street.

One Great Reason for Cutting Overseas Aid

One great reason for cutting overseas aid
is that this will make it harder
for poor countries to buy vaccines.
Then the illness and death rates will rise
in those countries
and it means the virus will remain
a constant threat in the world
as a whole.

Contagious

Reports coming in
that Conspiracy Theories
are highly contagious.

Take the usual precautions.

To Save People the Bother

I've commissioned a statue of myself
and when it's finished
I'll invite people to a statue-throwing party
and we'll throw it in the river.

Over in the Right-wing Mags

It's open war on the 'woke'.
All charitable motives must be doubted,
phony outrage expressed at anything
that smells of money-making
(as if the right oppose the acquisition of wealth!),
all agitation for justice to be ascribed to
undercover Bolshevism.

Being Jewish

There are keyboard warriors
who want to legislate
for who is or is not Jewish.
They find phrases to include and exclude:
hurdles to get over,
licences that need to be won
and then shown
whenever they demand it.
It works like Olympic high jumping:
the bar is raised knocking out people
who can't get over;
the difference being that in the Olympics
pushing the bar off
doesn't stop people calling you an athlete.
It has to be said
that in fact
there are no real legislators
in this matter.
Me being Jewish
is not decided by a Jewish pope
because there is no Jewish pope.
I just wander about being Jewish.
I wander about being a lot of things actually
and being Jewish is in there with the mix.
Then again, I'm not in a category like 'lapsed'.
I'm not a lapsed Jew.
I can't lapse.
I was just born that way.
I could always pretend I'm not
and possibly get away with it in some places
but someone would be bound to leak it.
Not that I'm trying.
But if you're peering over your glasses
and asking me
so what kind of Jew are you?

(because we all love a good category)
I could answer it by mentioning the Jews
I would like to be like.
Or a bit like.
Or like a bit of them.
Jews like Franz Kafka.
Joseph Heller, Lennie Bruce,
Walter Benjamin, Hannah Arendt, Sigmund Freud,
Rosa Luxembourg, Erich Fromm, Judith Kerr,
Karl Marx, Walter Matthau, Joan Rivers, Joe Slovo,
Larry David, Allen Ginsberg, Maurice Sendak
Jonathan Miller, Eve Merriam...
I won't go on.
That'll do me fine.
Oh but while I'm on,
here's two more:
Harold and Connie Rosen.

Sonnet for Anne Frank

Since you took us into that attic space
no room under the eaves has been the same.
Wherever we go – our homes or others
whenever we dip and duck under beams
you are in the shadows, writing pages
laughing, crying, eating, daring to love
imagining a better world than yours
How you wrote leads us to think we know you.

You compressed so much life into that loft
which we pore over and love you for it
yet the real world – not the one you imagined
didn't allow you to live and write anymore.
Each time we read, we struggle to enjoy
your love of life while knowing how it ended.

Learning

We are learning how to say
welcome
in Ukrainian.
Could we learn to say it in
some other languages too?

As If in a Dream

As if in a dream
I'm hearing radio programmes
playing Ukrainian patriotic songs
and lovingly produced discussions
about the history of Ukraine
and admiration pouring out of my radio and TV
for the brave people of Ukraine
daring to stand up to this terrible invasion
and I felt warm and sad at the same time
wrapped in the care and kindness of it all
and I was pouring out my admiration too,
and images from the TV came to me from last night
of hundreds of people squashed into a station subway
trying to get out on a train to Poland
and more sounds from the radio
of people on the border shivering and hungry and crying
not knowing if they could get out
while arcs of light flashed over apartment blocks
and the morning showed the cold grey ruins of people's homes
and I heard the words of sympathy
from our leaders
while they explained that Ukrainians
would need visas or relatives in Britain
if they want to come here
and I wasn't sure that people crushed
into the subway would have visas
or relatives here, would they?
so if they don't have visas and relatives
what happens to them in the freezing cold
on the Polish border?
and I thought about the care and kindness
coming out of my radio
and I felt uneasy
that I remember other invasions
other bombings,

and the same radio and TV stations
pouring out hours of words
on why similar bombings and invasions
were necessary and good bombings and invasions
and why those resisting were crazy and bad
and of course – as always –
why there wasn't room for people of those countries
to get out and come here
and I was left looking for the principle being defended here.
This principle can't be that it's wrong to invade
other countries.
The principle can't be that it's wrong
to bomb civilians.
The principle can't be that we must help
those who resist invasions.
The principle can't be that we must help
refugees.
But then I thought,
what's the matter with me?
what is the matter with me?
why am I looking for a principle?
Well, not a principle that lasts
or a principle that is valid in all places.
Our leaders' principles are things
they pick up, boast about
and then drop
in the hope that we can't remember anything
from before last week.
Or that we don't notice what else they do
in other parts of the world.
One moment they are friends with people
who are tyrants or backers of tyrants
and the next they are explaining to us
that the tyrants are tyrants
and friends of tyrants are the friends of tyrants
as if we didn't know that the tyrants are tyrants
and that they themselves are friends
with the friends of tyrants

as if we hadn't noticed this
as if we had now forgotten this.
And this is a cycle
that goes on and on turning,
it's turning in my mind
remembering my parents
talking of the leaders of their time
chumming up with Nazis
corporations selling oil to the Nazis
oil they would use to bomb us
and my parents talking of uncles and aunts and cousins
who criss-crossed the very same land
that the refugees are crossing now,
one who escaped
the rest who didn't
and it's a cycle
it's a cycle that grinds millions into the ground
burnt, dismembered, starved, maimed
and I am listening to the radio.
And I am listening to the radio.

If They Want To

There is a man on Newsnight
saying that the situation with refugees now
is different from when the UN drew up
its charter on refugee at the end of the
Second World War.
What could he have meant?

I switch channels.
The debate shifts to 'criminal gangs'.
Politicians who want to sound ethical
go on and on about criminal gangs.
The ethical thing to do with refugees is
to help them.
They could also make sure that they
don't bomb other countries.
And they could stop supplying arms
to governments that bomb other countries.
That is, if they really do want to save lives.

At the end of WW2,
the government hired boats
and brought the soldiers and thousands of refugees
who were them, to Britain.
Amongst them was my father's cousin.
They were put into Polish Resettlement Camps,
all over Britain.
I'm not saying it was perfect.
I'm not saying it was ideal.
There was all sorts of xenophobic
and racist stuff swirling about
but it remind us of what governments can do
if they want to.

Acknowledgements

'Renewal – a Soliloquy' was first broadcast on BBC Radio 2. 'Sonnet for Anne Frank' was commissioned by the Anne Frank Trust on the 75th anniversary of the publication of *Anne Frank's Diary*.